Looking After an Older Person

A Guide for Relatives and Friends

by

DEBBIE DRY
A Care Home Manager

CP
THE CHOIR PRESS

First published in the United Kingdom in 2023 by
The Choir Press

ISBN 978-1-78963-350-4

This book is dedicated to my mum and dad, Tom and Margaret, who always taught me to be kind to others.

Getting Old

Look at me now, all wrinkled and grey,
No one to talk to with nothing to say.
Left here abandoned, a man all alone,
Nowhere to go, I'm stuck in my home.

They used to come in here and tend to my love,
She is at rest now, in Heaven above.
We'd chat and laugh about a life worth living,
My love for the take and them for the giving.

But now I'm alone, for my loved one has flown,
Left me in jail or is it my home?
No one to talk to and no one to see,
Just memories, thoughts and silence for me.

As I do the routine in reverse at this time,
I long for the love and the life that was mine.
But time is a composer that cannot be won,
For I see my tomorrow, a new life has begun.

I yearn for the company of a heart and a voice,
I'd grasp it with haste, if given a choice.
Waiting for someone to knock on my door,
For death has no meaning, not for me any more.

AUTHOR

Contents

Part A
Getting Older

1.
Introduction

"To care is to do something; dignified care is to do it with meaning."   AUTHOR

Being able to care for someone and make a difference to their life is so rewarding. Often it can be the simplest acts that make the biggest impact. It has been my role as a care home manager that has provided me with the opportunity to spend time with wonderful individuals in their later years and towards the end of their lives. They shared some of their innermost thoughts and feelings, which they did not even share with family or friends. I was there not only to care for them but to listen and understand what they had to say. Some imparted knowledge about growing old, others explained that they had had enough of living and wanted to die, and there were those who did not see themselves as old and still wanted to enjoy life.

The information they shared shaped my attitude to this generation and the care I provided to help them live a meaningful life. With the input of their families, care staff and doctors, they were empowered to make decisions about what support and treatment they did and did not want, ensuring they had a voice and were treated with respect and dignity.

I decided to write a book about how to care for someone at this stage of their life because it can be a challenging time when a relative or friend becomes frail or deteriorates, requiring health or social care support. Social care can be complex, so this book is also to help navigate someone through the challenges that the health and social care system presents. It is also to highlight the different perspectives that an older person may have in relation to their abilities and how they are managing, and the perspective of those closest to them. Therefore, it is important at the beginning to establish effective communication and consider what the individual wants, and if indeed they even want any support or advice.

As people grow older and talk about their lives, they often refer to the different stages of growing up: childhood, being a young adult, family life and finally, getting older. As we age it seems natural to reflect on the life we have led and talk about the people or circumstances that have shaped who we are. We also bring to life memories of how we used to look, what we were doing at that time and who was in our life at that time. The more we age, the more we reminisce, because as we recall these memories, we recognise how quickly life moves on and how fragile life can be.

I have over 25 years' experience of caring for and living with older people. As a qualified nurse I have looked after people at their most vulnerable in hospital. I have also supported staff to provide person-centred care to people in the last stages of their lives and have witnessed many deaths over the years; and it is in those last moments of someone's life that you can provide the most sensitive, dignified care, observing the wishes of the person who is dying.

It has been in my role as a care home manager that I have learnt the most about caring holistically for a person. It has provided me with a valuable opportunity to observe individuals and to understand the physical, social and psychological impact that ageing has on them and their families. It has also enabled me to understand the unique relationship between the person who requires care and the person who supports them, be that a family member or a friend. Over the years I have been approached by family and friends of older people who have found the responsibility of looking after the well-being of an older person a daunting task. They have shared their experiences with me and expressed exasperation at the lack of guidance on how to care for someone else or how to arrange the care support that may be required.

This book is about using my knowledge and experience to help those who find themselves with the responsibility of caring for an older person and need guidance to facilitate them in arranging the best care for the individual.

With encouragement, this book aims to help the family or friends of someone who requires support put the interests and wishes of the individual at the forefront of all decision-making and enable them to be involved at every opportunity. It is also aimed at anyone who is considering living with an older relative and it will provide practical advice about care support and encourage the reader to contemplate the perspective of the older person and understand who they are now and what they are going through, physically and emotionally, at this stage of their life. This understanding will help facilitate a better appreciation of a person's behaviour and create a more mutual relationship between them both. For example, imagine a gentleman who has been independent all his life but after a sudden admission to hospital people are questioning whether he should return home. Supportive family members, health-care staff and social workers become involved and with the best intentions try to organise care provision, but they fail to step into the shoes of the gentleman. He becomes a mere observer of others making decisions about his life and where he should live. Often, as someone reaches a certain age, assumptions can be made about their capacity and ability without considering what they want or feel. In this example, with medication review, physiotherapy and minor adaptations to his home, this gentleman may still live happily and independently at home for many years. He may also decide to accept the consequences of returning home, putting him at risk of a fall or loneliness. While many do not understand this and want the individual to be safe, safety is not always the main concern as people become frail. Independence and having a say in how they spend their life and where they live is more important to them.

Looking after another adult is a huge responsibility, and to consider caring for someone else may cause people to question their involvement or motivation, such as, "Am I doing the right thing?", "What do I do now?" or "Who can I go to for help?" It may not only impact on the caring relative/advocate but also on their spouse or family, so it is important that you are honest with yourself about the level of support you can provide.

This book aims to assist family carers think about what options are available for someone in need of care support and where to access the help needed.

It is divided into 4 sections: Getting Older, Social-economic Factors, Activities of Daily Living and Support, focusing on ageing, funding, activities of daily living and, finally, sources of support. There are also some helpful tips within the chapters to consider, and Chapter 21 provides space to make notes or to document questions that arise as you read the book. It is also important to be clear about the role you want to play and what responsibilities you are ready to take on. Some people choose to be hands on and coordinate all care support, while others prefer to make enquiries on behalf of someone else and seek the guidance of a care agency or social services.

It is important to understand the complexity of caring for a person who is ageing. When one thinks of someone of a certain age or era, it is their physical state that first comes to mind, but their character, behaviour or attributes are rarely acknowledged. It is important, therefore, to look at the individual as a whole being. It is important to get to know the individual who exists now, rather than reflect on the person you think you know. Many times I have had a conversation with relatives telling me "She reads a lot" or "He never wears vests", yet after admission we learn that the lady hasn't read a book for a couple of years and the gentleman didn't wear vests when he was a young working man but as he has lost weight and feels the cold more he prefers to wear them. These are just two simple examples to show that with time people *do* naturally change their behaviour and attitudes, so it is important to not make assumptions.

Another factor to consider is the impact that loneliness and independence have on people as they age, and this may influence how they accept any well-meaning guidance or support from others. It is important to acknowledge that the advice from health-care professionals should always be considered but the preferences and wishes of the individual must take priority.

It is worth mentioning how important it is not to stereotype older people as a collective group, as the characters and personalities of older people vary, similar to any other age group when making an assessment. Older people can be portrayed as happy, joyful characters, similar to how grandparents are perceived, but they can also be stereotyped as grumpy, curmudgeonly characters like

Victor Meldrew in *One Foot in the Grave*, particularly some solitary characters. It is important not to judge or stereotype, and I personally believe that any aloofness or challenging behaviour usually indicates a fear of losing independence and control and is not a true reflection of the character within.

Therefore, before someone even begins the journey of helping to care for another adult, it is essential that they understand how the older generation are viewed by society, as this can influence the response that the person has when others become involved in their life. It will also highlight the challenges and preconceptions and ageism that some people must face and overcome on a regular basis.

Be prepared for the person to decline any support. It is worth having a conversation at this stage to acknowledge why the individual may prefer to be left alone. Is it because they are borne of a generation who do not want to cause a fuss and are quite happy how they are living their life? Even if someone declines support, it doesn't hurt to have the initial conversation about help that is available, so that they know there is support at a time when they feel they need it. A phone call or brief visit to an elderly relative or neighbour is also a wonderful opportunity to show you care.

Finally, by focusing on ageing and the impact this has on someone's life, it may cause the reader to reflect on their own thoughts and attitudes towards getting old and what their future could look like: retirement, illness, relationships, etc.

Each chapter is divided into themes to make it easier to navigate to the most relevant part of the book. It takes a holistic approach, looking at each person as an individual based on their physical, social and psychological well-being, to ultimately provide the best person-centred care for them.

Question:

Is there someone you know who needs support?

2.
Caring *About* or Caring *For* Someone

"We know what we are, but know not what we may be."

WILLIAM SHAKESPEARE

We all care *about* our family and relatives, but it is different to actually caring *for* them. This suggests more involvement and more responsibility. In my experience, many people take on the responsibility of caring for a family member suddenly, after an acute illness, recurrent falls or a hospital admission. When health-care professionals conclude the individual would be unlikely to manage at home alone and would require some care intervention, they contact family, or an advocate if there is no relative, to discuss discharge plans. It is crucial that the person who requires care is involved in all conversations and decisions that will affect their life. When returning home, a care package of support should be created. An occupational therapist (OT) would usually assess the home environment and provide new equipment or adapt it to make it safer. Carers could be arranged to visit several times daily to provide essential care needs. However, if it were deemed unsuitable or unsafe for a person to return home, there are other alternatives. There is more about alternative accommodation later in the book.

People may genuinely want the best for their relative or friend but may not be able to physically provide that care or the commitment that the role entails. It is a very hard decision to make, as caring about a family member, neighbour or friend is not the same as being their carer, so it is important to differentiate between the two.

Caring *about* someone refers to a strong feeling or affection for them but caring *for* someone, implies physically supporting their health needs and having responsibility for them. Whether you decide to coordinate the care support, research care accommodation or provide the care yourself will take time to deduce. There is no right or wrong in how to approach this, as each situation and person is unique. No one should feel overpowered or pressured into deciding this, as caring *about* another individual is just as important as caring *for* them.

Some family members may already be caring for a relative or friend but don't necessarily think of themselves as carers. They may have received no training for the role or payment for their involvement, but if they are looking after a relative, friend or partner who is ill or needs support, they are by definition a carer. Even popping round each week and checking someone has been eating and drinking or has newspapers regularly is caring. The role of a carer is someone who regularly looks after or assists someone in need, and it can be for any task, such as washing, social visits or shopping.

Being aware of what is happening in one's own life and the current commitments you have will also affect how you manage the situation and respond to being involved in someone else's care provision. When deciding to support someone in need, it is important to recognise that the relationship you currently have with them may alter – from caring *about* to caring *for* – and the person receiving this care will also need time to adapt to the change.

When people first enquire about a care home place on behalf of a relative, friend or neighbour, I always ask them the thoughts and opinions of the individual who may require a care home placement. I encourage relatives to bring the individual to the care home and experience it by observing and listening to what is happening during their visit; after all, no one considers buying a house on behalf of someone else, so why buy the services of a care home on behalf of someone else? This may become their home and they should be involved and experience the atmosphere of the place and meet the staff and the other residents. The ability to decide and make choices that affects them does not diminish with age. I also suggest they view a variety of establishments to make comparisons.

Place yourself in the older person's situation and ask yourself, "What if this was me?" This question underpins all decisions I make when caring for another person and encompasses the basic principles of care: privacy, dignity, rights, individuality, well-being, respect and choice. They embody the foundation of all care by ensuring that the person's needs always remain paramount in any situation.

Caring for an older person is complex. It can be difficult and challenging, but with the right advice and guidance it can also be rewarding and provide a sense of fulfilment in everyone's lives. It is important that everyone involved talks about the situation, expresses how they feel and are listened to when determining the best option for the person in need of care and companionship.

Question:

How well do you really know the person needing care?

3.
What Does It Feel Like to Be Ageing?

"Inside every old person is a young person wondering what happened."

TERRY PRATCHETT

In order to support someone who is ageing, it is important to consider how they feel and the physical, psychological and social impact that ageing may have on them. It is important to acknowledge the effect that age can have on a person, especially at a time where they may require minor support, as it may affect their sense of identity and overall well-being.

Each person is unique, but if people feel a loss of control in their lives, there is a possibility they may decline in overall health. Taking the right approach and supporting the individual to make decisions themselves keeps them in control and empowered to facilitate and dictate any changes that may occur within their lives.

So when someone says they need help or it appears they are not coping daily on their own, it is important to ask them what support they think they may need and how they feel about getting assistance from someone else. You may also tell them what help you feel they need and give examples of times you have felt they needed support, such as after a recent fall or if you have noticed they are not as socially engaged as they have previously been or they have not changed clothes in the last few days, which is unusual for them.

Deciding that they may need assistance, particularly for personal issues that they have managed all their life, is extremely difficult for someone to accept. The loss of control they feel and the acknowledgement that life (and age) is starting to affect how they live can be quite traumatic for people, and asking for help is also quite challenging. Therefore, it is important that, as the relative or friend of someone who is growing older, your approach to the situation is delicate and evolves over time.

Using the same terminology as health-care professionals is advantageous, as it breaks down a person's needs into categories. Activities of daily living (ADLs) is a term used in health care that provides a guide to identify someone's ability to care for themselves or highlights any need for support. This typically includes personal care, mobility, sleeping, social interactions, etc. Overall, it creates a picture or evidence of how well someone is managing daily. The greater the dependency in activities of living, the more care an individual is likely to require.

Loss of independence is closely associated with high dependency and this can be quite traumatic for an individual. Imagine living alone and living independently for most of your life and suddenly, as you become older and frailer, people close to you or a health-care professional start making decisions about where you live, how you should live and what care support you need.

Although people act with the best intentions, some do not talk to the individual, as asking someone how they are managing or raising any concerns they may have can be a difficult topic to approach. This is more evident in hospital, when a quick discharge is sought to free hospital beds and not enough time is given to the possible psychological ramifications on an ageing person. The earlier this conversation takes place, the better. I often ask residents in my care home how they feel they are managing and if they would like more support, as it provides them with an opportunity to tell me how they feel and encourages me to look at our care provision from their perspective.

It's important to observe the process of ageing rather than the fact of being old. We all have different ideas of what age a person is considered old and this affects how they are perceived and treated. A continuous reference to age – elderly, older person or geriatric – may cause offense and create a stereotype of someone elderly because of their chronological age, with no reference to their physical abilities, employment status or outlook on life. Many people are still in employment after retirement age and are extremely active, both socially and physically.

The quality of life for older people has dramatically improved over the past few decades. They have greater financial stability and are living longer and healthier lives. It is therefore certain that as life expectancy increases, the definition of old age will also alter. Centuries ago, the life expectancy of a man was 50 and this was therefore considered old. Now it is 79 years of age. As life expectancy increases, people currently in their sixties may be considered middle-aged in the future. It is something worth considering and is important because it will influence our attitudes to people within certain age groups, which also often reflects how they perceive themselves. For example, if someone keeps telling you that you are too frail and cannot manage, you will start to act that way and give up. ("Why bother trying? They don't believe me.") If you are at an age where you feel you have had enough of life, this can affect your attitude to living.

In our care home we had a lady who had a very clear sense of identity and of where she was in her life journey but she felt she was a burden on her daughter. At 99 years of age, she felt she had "had enough of life". What was important to her was for her daughter to live her own life instead of visiting her each day. Each night when staff said goodnight to this lady and told her they would see her in the morning, she used to reply "I hope not, dear", explaining that she hoped she would just close her eyes and not wake up. Staff found this distressing at first, but after asking the lady to explain, I began to understand her feelings. She had a complex medical history and at 99 years of age her quality of life (in her words) was not as good as it had been, and for many years she found this difficult to accept. Her life was not meaningful to her; although everyone showed her care and attention, it was not what she wanted any more. She felt she was existing and not living.

This contrasted with another lady who resided in our home. She was admitted from hospital following a fall at home and had been lying on the floor for eight hours, unable to reach her alarm bell. After a couple of weeks, hospital staff and her family concluded that she could no longer manage at home, but the lady wanted to go home, where she had lived for over 50 years. Her family and the medical staff felt she was not safe to live at home, but she was adamant she wanted to go home. She was reluctant to have carers but eventually agreed. She also agreed to a period of convalescence in our care home, where she stayed for eight weeks. During this time her mobility improved, her weight increased slowly and she socialised regularly with other residents. Although she said she loved her time with us, she wasn't ready to go into a care home. I had to agree with her. Home is more than just a building; a person's life story and family memories reside there. In fact, it became evident that she was 'not yet ready' for a care home at this stage. Therefore, it is important not to jump to any conclusions, and a regular assessment of an individual's abilities and need for assistance should be completed before deciding on a care home placement or alternative accommodation. A care home may be the right option in the future.

When a health-care professional makes an assessment about an individual, they observe someone by looking for different signs to make a judgement about the perceived quality of life. Obviously, they will take into account the person's chronological age, but this will only be for reference and will not usually determine the outcome of an assessment. They will also observe any slowing down in physical or mental agility, as well as a decrease in social interaction or activities in general. They will also consider any diagnosis such as Parkinson's or a stroke, number of recent falls or hospital admissions. Their outcome may be influenced by a frailty score, which measures a person's level of vulnerability. It assists the health-care profession with creating an overall picture of an individual's possible needs and, therefore, how to help manage someone's health.

The problem with this is that it predominantly reflects the physical abilities of someone rather than the cognitive or social aspects (although they are mentioned). This assessment also usually takes place at a time when someone is at their most vulnerable and are usually getting over an illness or acute episode, so it can be a snapshot of level of frailty rather than an accurate assessment of overall need.

Question:

What does the person really want and how can you help?

4.
The Three Ages of Ageing: Knowing, Feeling and Looking

"Age is no barrier to care."   Author

Often society can become fixated on a person's chronological age and make assumptions about their abilities and cognitive function. This is more evident in people who are ageing, and a common misconception is that everyone becomes hard of hearing as they age, but this is not true; some just need to filter noises and pitches that may be occurring at the same time, as these can be a distraction. We are all guilty of talking to a grandparent while we are facing away from them or while they are trying to listen to the radio or TV. By merely waiting for acoustic noise to subside and speaking clearly, facing them, we can enable them to hear perfectly well. So it is a fault in the talking process of the communication rather than the listening.

When I care or support someone, I ask them to reflect on their overall well-being at this stage in their life. By asking them their age, how old they feel and how old they think they look, I am provided with some insight into how they perceive themselves and how well they are living their life. Often it will encourage them to expand: "I'm 98 but I still feel as if I'm only in my seventies" or "I know I don't look like I used to, but I'm still with it". Even Sir Bruce Forsyth declared he still felt 30 years of age when he went on stage, even though he was 85 at the time. How others respond to this can also impact on the individual. It is therefore important to ask these questions and use the information to assist in how you approach someone who may require care support.

I have noted over the years that after a certain age people rarely look in the mirror. In our care home there are mirrors everywhere: in the lounge, corridors, bathrooms, kitchen and in each resident's room. Rarely do any of the residents choose to look in the mirror or ask to see themselves in one. This is either because they don't want to or they don't see it as part of their routine and are comfortable with how they feel and look. There are some individuals who still prefer to retain the image they have of themselves from years ago rather than the reflection they see in the mirror. This is relevant, as a person may only feel old when someone highlights the fact that they appear frail or are not managing. In essence, if someone does not want to feel old, it is easier to decline any offer of assistance, both from social services or a kind relative or neighbour. But how are older people meant to react when someone declares they are not managing or suggests they may need assistance when they feel they are managing rather well? After all, we are all different and lead our lives differently. Some people are considered old in chronological age but may display youthful characteristics, and others are younger but, due to illness or other factors, may appear frailer.

When we look at our own lives, we can subconsciously relate to our age in different ways: how old we are, how old we feel and how old we view ourselves. I believe this is true for any adult.

If an older person is having a good day, is socially aware and is involved in what is happening around them, they are more likely to say they feel younger than their real age. However, if they are lonely or have no social stimuli, they may say they feel old, and this in turn can impact on how they view care support and their willingness to accept it. This has always intrigued me, so I wanted to test the perception of age.

I asked a group of care home residents, all of whom were over 80 years of age, how old they were and how old they felt on a particular day. One lady declared she felt she was in her sixties, although she and I knew she would turn 95 on her next birthday. Each person stated that they did not feel their age, and the age they felt was irrelevant; what *was* important was that they all felt younger than their actual age. Most replied that they felt no different to how they felt in their twenties and thirties. However, they also acknowledged that they were not able to do things now that they were able to do when they were younger. This was important when understanding how to address each individual and how they responded to care support.

They also recalled that when they were children they rarely heard of anyone living beyond their nineties and the thought of anyone reaching 100 years of age sounded scarcely credible for their generation.

Personally, I believe the chronological age for an individual is not important. What is relevant is what age they *feel* they are, as it impacts on their behaviour and attitude, and while physical and psychological aging are interlinked, a person may describe an age they feel physically but identify a different age psychologically. This may be because frailty has made a visible and physical impact on their body but psychologically they describe themselves as feeling the same as they did when they were in their thirties or forties. After all, it is often said in society today that 60 is the new 40! However, for society and health-care planners, it is important to identify actual ages, as frailty and diagnoses and implications of illness or disease will have an impact on health and social care and the financial cost of care provision for now and future planning.

As a society we sometimes become too concerned about the age of an individual. In hospital, if someone is over 90, health-care professionals are more likely to consider limited treatment or the decision not to admit to an intensive-care unit, or have a 'do not attempt cardiopulmonary resuscitation' (DNACPR) order added to those individuals, based on their diagnosis but influenced by their chronological age. This disregards their quality of life or overall well-being. Of course, the diagnosis of a terminal illness or non-response to conventional treatment could influence the discussions and the decision being made, but a life is a life, and the individual and their family should always be consulted.

In essence, when consulting someone about needing care, it is important to ask them their chronological age and the age they feel. This may have an impact on the decisions they make and influence any acceptance of care and the approach you take.

Question:

How old does the person feel?

5.
The Psychological Impact of Ageing

"They don't care what you know; they want to know that you care." ANON

Growing old is inevitable for everyone and is a natural progression of living, but there is usually an impetus that causes us to re-evaluate our lives and think about our future and the life we have left. It may be the result of a change in ourselves or those around us or the death of a family member, as how we grow old can be influenced by our attitudes, experiences in life and people who have influenced us.

We have already explored in Chapter 3 what it feels like to be ageing but this chapter is concerned with the emotional and mental state of ageing. This can influence someone's behaviour or attitude and how they decide to live the rest of their life.

We all reach milestones throughout life. Teenagers are deemed as approaching adulthood and at 18 years of age they legally become an adult. By the age of 21 people have usually set out on their career pathway or are studying at a higher education institution. They are less likely to be dependent on family and are making their own way in the world. Certain ages depict stages of life and periods of getting older and can be met with a mixture of emotions, both positive and negative. I had a friend who panicked at the age of 25, and when I asked her why (as I had no problem with it; I was still young), she replied that she had lived a quarter of a century already and had not really done anything. In reality, she had trained as a nurse for three and a half years and was working well within the profession.

What happens after 50 can depend on the individual, their

attitude to life and their social network. Sometimes it can be the age itself that alters a person's attitude to getting older (as in my friend's example) or a new decade – 40 or 50 years of age – and for others illness or disease may be the catalyst to force people to reflect and re-evaluate their lives. This can occur at any age, not just older life.

Retirement

The attitude that an individual has to life in general can impact on their sense of self and well-being. Many view post-retirement as a time of slowing down, with less financial worries and more time to be free of any constraints, but others may feel a sense of loss, no longer being part of the wider community and workforce. How people react to retirement and spend their time can affect how they enter the later stages of life. I have met many people who have come into our care home and have spent retirement remaining active within their community or maintaining close links with family and friends. Nevertheless, I have also cared for individuals who have spent the majority of their lives alone, at home, without talking or engaging with others regularly, and over many years this can affect their confidence and self-esteem.

It is therefore essential that health-care professionals, family members and those involved in organising care for an older person should focus on the whole person. In my experience, the physical, social and mental well-being of an individual are all closely aligned and must all be considered for the real understanding of a person and to facilitate a holistic, person-centred approach to their care.

Attitude and Behaviour

People require care for a variety of reasons. It may be for a short-term period, such as post-operative discharge from hospital, after a fall at home or long-term care after a diagnosis of illness or frailty. How they react to the challenges and how people support or interact with them is very significant and can influence the behaviour of the individual. Valuing them is crucial, and they should be empowered to embrace older age and to approach it with courage.

However, the impact of an acute change in someone who is older cannot be underestimated. This was more evident to me when we had a couple admitted into our care home. They were alert and physically able but were very dependent on each other. The lady was the more dominant character and answered most of the questions directed to them as a couple. They had been married for over 50 years when they came into the home. The reason they came into a care home, as the wife explained, was because she was due to have planned surgery within the next year and she wanted to settle her husband into a care home, so she knew he would be well looked after should anything go wrong with her operation.

The night before she went into hospital, she was very relaxed, and after her husband went to bed she calmly told staff she did not think she would survive the operation but she felt happy she had found a good home for her husband. Staff tried to reassure her that everything would be fine and that everyone becomes nervous before an operation and not to worry. Her husband would be looked after and staff would visit her after the operation. Yet she was so adamant that she would not survive, despite the reassurance of staff.

Unfortunately, this lady was right and she sadly had operative complications and passed away soon after surgery. Her husband was informed by a family member, with extra staff called in to support him, and for each other, as it was a shock for everyone. He was obviously distraught, but what you could not have foreseen was the psychological impact that grief and shock had on him.

Almost overnight he became unsettled, incontinent and confused. He seemed so lost, as though life meant nothing to him any more, as she was no longer around. He would wander around the garden talking to himself or to her memory. It was so sad to see, because even though he had been emotionally dependent on her, he physically and mentally deteriorated almost overnight when he heard she had died. He remained this way for many weeks and never really recovered, ageing quickly, eating less and becoming more dependent on others and neglecting himself, refusing to wash, shave or engage with anyone. Physically, he had been a strong gentleman, over six foot, but psychologically he became frail and emotionally dependent. No one should underestimate the impact that losing a loved one has on an individual, particularly when there is an existing dependency.

One reason I love my job is because people intrigue me, and some people you meet within care, whether in hospital or a care home, have lived extraordinary lives. Once you learn the history of an individual and the life they have led, it equips you with the narrative to understand the individual you care about and how the influences and challenges they have encountered during their life have helped shape them.

As a society, how we view and treat older people reflects the perception we have of growing old and this will influence the next generation. It is important that those who are in a privileged position to influence society and their local communities start changing the stereotypical view of an older person and highlight the positives of getting older and the positive contribution older people make to society. Older people can be role models: for instance Sir Tom Jones, Dame Judi Dench and Dame Joan Bakewell. They always look great, are vibrant, contribute to society and are confident, wise and funny.

Loneliness

Over the past 20 years of being a care home manager, I have become more concerned with the increasing number of people who enter care homes on antidepressants or mood-stabilising medication. While I do not know the reason some of them were started on them initially, it has become more obvious that years of living alone and feeling lonely may have caused them to become depressed. Years of remaining on this medication may not be beneficial for them and they should be reviewed regularly by a medical practitioner.

I have also observed individuals transform after being in a care home and beginning to socialise and engage with others and improve their quality of life. One lady, who had lived alone for 15 years after her partner had died and had been with us for a few months, declared, "I never realised how lonely I was until I came here." She had made friends and socialised with staff and other residents and, most importantly, had something to look forward to each day.

Loneliness can manifest in different ways – paranoia, depression or being withdrawn – and anyone who is frail many feel trapped in their own home. A recent poll has shown that the majority of respondents said that their close friends and family would be surprised or astonished to hear that they felt lonely. It is something people do not talk about or usually admit to.

In 2017 Age UK found that people over the age of 50 were more likely to be lonely if they:

- had no one to open up to
- were widowed
- were in poor health
- felt as if they did not belong in the neighbourhood
- were unable to do what they wanted
- lived alone

However, it is important not to assume that everyone who lives alone is lonely. Many people prefer their own company and engage with others when they choose to or when the opportunity arises. We have all learnt more recently that technology has been a fantastic lifesaver for many people who live alone, and using social media platforms to communicate with family members has improved their well-being and socialisation. This may be something to consider if someone lives alone – adding apps or videos onto an iPad or computer – as it may improve an older person's socialisation. Nowadays people do not need to physically meet to socialise, and, therefore, this option should be explored.

It is important to talk to the individual and observe how they spend their day (activities and socialisation), how often they can talk to people and if they have any interests or hobbies. These are questions we ask when someone is interested in a care home placement as it gives us insight into the well-being of an individual.

Question:

Does the person appear lonely?

What Loneliness Saw

There he is, that same man, still staring are we;
I do not recognise him, yet he seems to know me.
He appears again unshaven, with no sense of pride;
I call out to reach him, but cowering, he hides.

I see him here most days, alone and forlorn;
I want to speak up, but my conscience is torn.
He makes me feel eerie, his presence each day;
No expression, no meaning, with nothing to say.
Just watching my moves, he stares only ahead;
I can't take it much more, "Enough!" I said.
"Why do you follow? Why not leave me alone?"
"Why are you here again? This is MY home."

The anger distorts me, my rage in despair,
But the figure I notice, the same features we share.
His anger appears greater and more threatening than me,
But as I go nearer, his outlines I see.
That old man's no stranger ... That old man IS ME!

There in the mirror we stand faced at last;
United in grief, we recall our past.
What's happened to us? Where did it go wrong?
Closing our eyes, for the memory that's gone.
Our thoughts mill together, expressed in a sigh,
And together for a moment, we recall days gone by.

How times have changed; we used to be free
To think for ourselves and do as we please.
We'd wash, dress and ready to face daily chores,
And to meet likewise people was never a bore.
But that has now changed, it's so plain to see,
How that old man there stopped me living AS ME!

I watch with intense as he mimics my being;
He stares and waits and it's then I start seeing
the chance to change and take all control
Of my life again, feel alive and feel whole.

With a wipe and a smear, I remove him from view
Another chance at life, to be the man I once knew.
To live and exist in the world that's outside,
I smile and turn around, for no more I'll hide.
My spine straightens up and my lungs do expand
To reflect the new vigour my body commands.
The feeling of life limbers through me, whole,
Deciding to live with my heart and my soul.

AUTHOR

Part B
Social-economic Factors

6.
Society and How We Treat the Elderly

"A test of people is how it behaves towards the old. It is easy to love children. Even tyrants and dictators make a point of being fond of children. But the affection and care for the old, the incurable, the helpless, are the true gold mines of a culture."

ABRAHAM J. HESCHEL

There are now 11.8 million people aged 65 or over in the UK, almost a third of whom live alone. That is over three and a half million people living alone. Years ago, most older relatives were looked after in the family home and cared for by family members, but over the last couple of decades the traditional nuclear family has declined in the modern world. This has impacted on the values and views we hold as a society on many aspects of life, such as money, family and community, and this in turn influences the opinion held of older people in society.

Why is this important, you may ask. It is important because the behaviour of someone as they grow older can be influenced by how they have been treated and viewed by the community around them and society at large, either personally or by the media. This can impact on any support or advice that is offered to them at a later stage. Sixty per cent of older people in the UK agree that age discrimination exists in the daily lives of older people.

As one of the most vulnerable groups in society, older people can be viewed as an inconvenience on top of the everyday pressures of life: working parents, childcare, mortgage and time constraints. When visiting a care home, relatives usually declare, "I couldn't possibly look after my mother/father/aunt. I have my own family." Therefore, they are perceived as a 'plus one' and not considered part of the family. This is very different from the traditional views of parents and grandparents in previous generations. That is not to say that anyone should feel guilty, but as people are living longer, maybe it is something that should be considered in the future when building houses or communities.

There are many benefits from engaging with someone of a different generation. I have had the opportunity to talk to many people after they have retired and come into our care home who have reminisced about their life experiences, such as taking the train to Trafalgar Square on D-Day, and performing in the theatre in London at the annual Harrod's staff end-of-year show. Another resident would cycle six miles daily to the local shop and put her shopping in her small basket. She continued this even in her seventies.

When local school children visit to sing or take part in craft workshops with residents, it is wonderful to hear them laugh and tell stories of a time that is so different to the world we currently live in.

Some relatives may be unable to care for a family member, as they feel out of their depth or unprepared for the role, and this is totally understandable. The role they can play is in helping the person navigate aspects of care provision that are available and help to choose the one most appropriate for their needs. This may change over time, so someone who opts to have carers visit once or twice a day may later choose to receive additional support or move to supported-living accommodation. This doesn't mean the family member is expected to deliver or coordinate their care but can be an advocate for the individual, to promote the involvement of the individual and acknowledge their wishes.

Periodically telephoning or visiting a relative to see how they are, or having grandchildren telephone or write, is also an opportunity to have a conversation to facilitate the individual to talk about what they have been doing and if they need anything. This reassures them that someone cares about them. It can be very enlightening and can provide some insight into how the person feels and how they are managing.

Technology is a great tool to enable instant connection using various formats of iPads and phones at the touch of a button. With many technological advances, people are able to safely remain in their homes for longer and from my experience this is more preferable for the individual.

Therefore, as the number of older people continues to increase, as it has over the last 50 years, society needs to modernise its view on people and end any biased views of a tired, slow generation. Look at the examples of Sir Ian McKellen and Dame Maggie Smith, who are over 80 years of age yet are strong, independent characters, who are still as busy now as they were 30 years ago.

We are trying to raise the profile of people who live in care homes and invite the community to engage with and visit people within the home. Working with local schools in an inter-generational project encourages children and older people to meet and share experiences, to talk to each other and bridge the age gap. It has been a fantastic opportunity for the two generations to be creative together and to listen to the issues that concern them both.

Others who promote older life and provide advice to older people should also continue to play their part in promoting a positive later life. Age UK, a charity designed to support older people in life, encourages older people to love later life and live it to the full. They often use the services of a celebrity ambassador to promote the message and the work they stand for. This is great, as any message raising the profile of the older generation must be recognised and commended.

However, I would also welcome the promotion of the great care that is already happening in the community. During the Covid-19 pandemic, where care homes were instructed to receive people discharged from hospital who'd tested positive to Covid, without health-care support or supplies of personal protective equipment (PPE), the lack of knowledge and awareness of the great work that care staff contribute to the community was demonstrated.

Question:

How do you treat older people?

7.
The Right Care Environment

"He is happiest, be he king or peasant, who finds peace in his home"

JOHANN WOLFGANG VON GOETHE

There will come a time when an individual and those involved with their care and well-being will question whether the person requires a greater level of care than can be provided at home. The person may need long-term care, such as that provided in a care home or sheltered housing. This can be a very difficult and emotional time for them, as it involves a huge change in their life. Home is more than the bricks of a building; it is the memories and the life led within it.

Entering the social-care system can be complex, so it is wise to ask social services for a care assessment at this point and to get advice from those who have knowledge of the care services and care system. The assessment can be completed by social services, who will decide the level of care required based on the individual's needs and whether they are entitled to any financial support. Most local councils have the same criteria to determine who is entitled to social care. There are many different care providers and standards of care provided, so it is important to choose the right one.

Moving into any care establishment is a huge experience and change in someone's life. It is important that they are involved at all stages of the transition and decide themselves whether receiving care in their own home or moving into a care environment is right for them. Families and advocates must act with integrity, as the impact of change and an individual's involvement in the process will adversely affect the person both physically and psychologically.

As well as social services, the local library also has resources to guide people to care-support options, but many people rely on word of mouth, especially if they have had positive experiences from care services. It is worthwhile researching all positive care provisions that may be referred to you, either through word of mouth or by visiting the Care Quality Commission (CQC) website to review inspection reports.

The CQC is the care regulator, and evidence from its reviews show that standards of care overall are improving over time. Although there is still a long way to go, the majority of care managers across the industry want the best for the people in their care.

Many care providers are specifically designed to care for people with a diagnosis of dementia, but a care home is not always the best option. Some people with dementia do have the capacity to make decisions about where they wish to reside and what care support they require. They should also be encouraged to remain involved in any decisions about their care, if possible. As people's care needs alter and their level of dependency increases, they may require extra support or 24-hour care, so it is important to seek extra support each time someone's dependency level changes and when researching different care provisions.

Helpful Tip

It is worth observing and documenting how much care the individual requires (Chapter 21 is available for this). Make notes on how they spend their day, how they mobilise or how often they get up to go to the toilet at night. Do they make their own meals or do they rely on others? Are they independent or do they have assistance regularly? This information will be crucial to share with providers of care, as it will provide an honest account of someone's independence and level of need. It will help everyone understand what level of support an individual requires.

There is also funding guidance in Chapter 18, as this is another complex area where further advice from social services or a solicitor may be required.

Different Care Provisions

In the community there are also options for care services to assist an individual to live as independently as possible at home, such as home meal delivery, telecare home alarm systems and day centres. These vary greatly, even within the same county, so check with social services for more information.

Other care providers include:

Domiciliary Care – This is care provided by an agency in the community. The carer will go into an individual's home to provide the help that has been agreed, such as personal care, shopping and serving meals. Visits can vary from half an hour to a few hours and this is negotiated with the domiciliary care provider.

Live-in carer – This is when a carer is paid to live with the individual in their own home and care for their needs, including personal care, shopping, cooking and companionship. They would need to be provided with a room of their own in the accommodation. It is important when employing a carer that they have been through thorough checks, including references and a safeguarding Disclosure and Barring (DBS) check. If employing someone from an agency, it is important to ask for confirmation of these basic checks.

Sheltered accommodation – This is for someone who is still relatively independent but can no longer manage at home alone. A flat or room can be bought or rented in a sheltered-housing complex. A warden is usually on-site during the day and there are other people in similar circumstances living there. A communal lounge is also available. It is often viewed as a halfway between home and a residential care home.

Care Village – These are becoming popular and are similar to sheltered housing but are usually larger with facilities on site, such as shops and hairdressers; some even have gyms, cafés and a doctor's surgery. They have communal areas and activities during the day but these can be more expensive.

Residential care – This is a care home that provides care and accommodation similar to a nursing home but the individual is still relatively active and independent. They may still require assistance with personal care, washing, dressing and mobility. Some residential care homes also take individuals requiring catheters, stomas or oxygen. The level of support varies within each care home, depending on their registration, environment and resources.

Nursing care – If you are a resident in a nursing home, and you have been assessed as requiring the services of a nurse, NHS-funded nursing care can be paid directly to the nursing home at a standard and higher rate.

Respite Care – If a family member/carer provides care for an older person and they need a break, some care homes have rooms that provide short-term care for an individual while their primary carer is away. This can be for a few days and up to a month. It can also be used as an opportunity for the older person to trial a period of time in a care home. For some people it confirms they are not yet ready to go into a care home long term, and others they enjoy the experience so much they decide to remain.

Living with Family – For some, the thought of placing their loved one into a care home is not an option and they may ask their relative to move in with them, either adapting their home or adding an extension/self-contained flat. This multigenerational concept is not new, as in many cultures it is just assumed that older generations will be cared for by their younger family members.

> *Question:*
>
> *Does the individual want to remain where they are living?*

8.
Safeguarding

"In order for evil to flourish, all that is required is for good men to do nothing."

EDWARD BURKE

The safety and welfare of a person who is vulnerable or in need of care support is paramount. It is essential that all decisions are risk-assessed to ensure that the right decision is made and that the individual is not placed at any risk. There is a balance between ensuring the person is safe and enabling them to make decisions, even if you do not agree with them. The challenge is that, with good intentions, people can be overly cautious and inevitably make what they feel is the *safest* option rather than what is the *right* option for the individual at that time.

Therefore, it is important to encourage or empower the individual to speak up and to explain what support they feel they may need. This message is consistently promoted throughout the book. It can be reassuring for the individual to know that a family member or friend will act as a support or advocate for them and will not force any decisions on them. This can be more evident when liaising with social services or care providers, as they often have time constraints and prefer quick decisions to be made. They may also use unfamiliar terminology, which is not always understood by people outside of the health and social-care professions.

You may be embarking on a journey of seeking care support, where you will research different care agencies and establishments. A list of registered services is available in all social services departments, council offices, community libraries and the CQC website. As mentioned previously, the CQC is the regulator for providers of health and care services. Their website will provide you with inspection reports and provide insight into the quality of care provided (at a given time) by each registered provider (www.cqc.org.uk).

There should also be information on each care agency or establishment's website explaining the service they provide, their aims and objectives, their complaints procedure and their quality assurance practices. It is essential that there is always a statement of recognition for the safety and welfare of all vulnerable people in their care, as this provides a sense of recognition and awareness that safeguarding is a fundamental focus within their organisation.

Over the decades, care homes have predominantly been portrayed as uncaring and poorly managed institutions, especially over the last ten years, where examples of appalling care homes have been scrutinised. In 2014 a *Panorama* TV programme highlighted the neglect and abuse of vulnerable people, focusing mainly on care homes. I watched the programme in horror, and disbelief that this was occurring in modern society and within my own profession. Although I applaud the programme makers for highlighting this issue, I feel more research behind the story was needed. Rather than just identifying the perpetrators, there should have been more investigation behind the culture and management of each establishment. It is important to discover who monitored standards of care, how the abuse was ever tolerated in each establishment, how long the abuse went on for and why nobody did anything about it. I would hope the examples used in this programme reflect only a handful of perpetrators, who should never have been allowed to look after vulnerable individuals.

Safeguarding is everyone's business, regardless of whether the person is at home or in receipt of care from an external agency. Abuse can happen anywhere, in care and at home, usually by people known to the victim. In fact, many cases of abuse, particularly financial abuse, occurs within the individual's own home. The safety and welfare of all individuals receiving care or support is the priority. The culture of keeping quiet and doing nothing for fear of reprisals must end! Each council has a safeguarding board to respond quickly to any concerns of abuse, but they are also available for guidance and support if you believe someone is at risk.

It is totally unacceptable for any member of staff to be aware of poor standards of care or abuse and do nothing about it. This is a more widespread problem and does not just stop with the abuser; it extends to every member of staff who continues to work in any care organisation and yet remains silent. The Care Act (2014) standards state that all staff should receive an induction programme and be trained in the duty of care and safeguarding.

There are so many opportunities for staff to raise concerns about poor attitudes or poor quality of care and inform others – such as supervisors, senior managers, CQC, social services, proprietors or the board of trustees of a care service – or even voice concerns to a colleague. The CQC website makes it easy to raise a concern regarding any type of abuse online and to the local safeguarding team within the county council.

All care establishments and agencies should have whistle-blowing and safeguarding policies to protect both the vulnerable and the whistle-blower from any repercussions. Any tool that encourages staff to speak up to protect the well-being of all vulnerable people should be entrenched in all induction and training programmes for new and long-term staff members. Whistleblowing in care can be a frightening prospect for some staff, for fear of reprisals, especially as there have been some high-profile cases in the media where people have lost their jobs in the National Health Service (NHS) for raising concerns. I would question whether these were true issues of whistleblowing or a conspiracy of NHS establishments in covering up systemic failures. People must learn to take responsibility for their actions or lack of action.

I can wholeheartedly declare that if I saw any mistreatment, poor standards of care or abuse, I would report my concerns with no hesitation, even if it meant upsetting colleagues or even losing my job. It comes back to the kind of person you are and the qualities and values that guide you throughout life. The people in my care come first and this should be taught and practised in every care agency and establishment.

More families are choosing to install CCTV in the private homes of relatives who receive care. This is also a wise option, but it is worth researching the legal implications of this, as carers in the course of their employment also have rights and consent must be sought from the owner of the property before CCTV can be installed within their property.

Question:

Do you have any safeguarding concerns?

9.
Socialisation

"There is no greater disability in society, than the inability to see a person as more."

ROBERT M. HENSEL

As humans, it is in our nature to want to spend time with others: to chat to, to share experiences with and to learn from. Just because people age, doesn't mean they lose this basic need. Without social interaction, isolation, loneliness and depression can become embedded quite quickly. When older people socialise, their quality of life is generally improved. It is important to know how the person likes to spend their day and to promote an active mind and body. There are numerous studies promoting regular exercise as a way of preventing physical and overall decline in well-being.

Community gives us a sense of belonging and being part of society. Years ago people were likely to know their neighbours, local shopkeepers and post office staff. A visit to any of these places offered a lifeline to many, as it was more than just buying groceries; it was also a quick chat of companionship and friendship. Over the years, this has changed dramatically, as towns have expanded and people move for work or housing opportunities. Transportation within a community setting also has an impact on the socialisation of someone who is over retirement age. Therefore, many must rely on family, good neighbours or teams of volunteers from community or faith groups for free transportation, without whom many would spend days without any social contact.

Helpful Tips for Socialisation:

- Exercise at home or join a local health club (there are initiatives for retirees and cost savings for membership).
- Go outside regularly – library, shops, garden centres, etc.
- Have the radio or TV on in the house (company).
- Have visitors – planned visits, especially from grandchildren.
- Complete puzzles, crosswords or sudoku books. They are good for mental health.
- Use newspapers and television planners to plan or record programmes to watch.
- Have plants in the house to provide tranquillity.
- Start or continue a hobby – join a craft group or reading club.

When someone moves into a care home, they are encouraged to invite relatives, friends and neighbours to continue visiting, and to continue with any social events or day centres they attend. This helps maintain their community and family links. However, care homes also employ activity coordinators who ensure that a variety of activities are arranged during the week. Residents are also encouraged to get involved with the functions within the home, such as interviewing potential new staff, choosing décor within the home and contributing to the regular newsletters and blogs on websites. They can also attend meetings within the county as representatives of the care home. Keeping the mind and body active has shown to help prevent illness and disease in later life.

We admitted a lady into our home who did not socialise. She had lived on her own all her life, having never married or had children. Over time she felt comfortable joining in activities with other residents and staff. Some days she still prefers being on her own and other days she decides when she wants to join in with other residents. This is fine, and five years later she remains in control. She has often thanked staff for making her feel part of a family, something she unfortunately never had the opportunity of experiencing before in her adult life, and she will soon reach her centenary birthday!

Activities/Hobbies

The hobbies and interests of each individual should be acknowledged so that they are encouraged to continue with pursuits or start something new and, therefore, have events they can look forward to. Some rely on weekly planners or calendars so they can plan activities at a pace they prefer.

It is also worth investing in the right technology and protecting people from any online scams. Older people are vulnerable to scammers, particularly hard-luck stories. We often tell residents, "If it's too good to be true, it probably is." Therefore, it is worth checking the security of any tablets that the individual may use and downloading antivirus software.

Trust and Friendship

Friendships can last over decades and can be valued more than any material possession. Family members are of course vitally important, but friends share a special bond. They are likely to be of the same generation, sharing similar experiences, memories or values and attitudes to life.

Be aware of any recent friendships that the individual has made. Of course, it is unfair to tarnish everyone with the same brush, but, nonetheless, there are people who take advantage of older people who live alone or are frail. We had one lady who inherited a vast amount of money, and soon after she moved in a gentleman friend of hers would visit. At first we thought nothing of it. He was pleasant and she enjoyed his company, but he was a married man and approximately 30 to 40 years younger than her. Staff noticed that he would kiss her hand and tell her how lovely she looked (at 92 she did look remarkable for her age). This lady was mesmerised and infatuated with him. He would take her out for dinner, but she always paid, and staff noticed she always brought her cheque book on these outings. However, he made staff feel uncomfortable and everyone was concerned she was being hoodwinked by him, so we called the local safeguarding team at the council for advice. They investigated our concerns but explained that as this lady had the capacity to decide what to do with her money (even though the circumstances were suspicious), there was nothing that could be done. The bottom line was that she gave her consent for him to have her money and she treated him to meals, as she enjoyed his company and he made her feel happy. It was a difficult situation but we had to accept that, in effect, she was paying for his companionship and it made her feel good.

Again, providing a calendar or diary for someone to write any events, outings or visits is a great way for individuals to plan their weeks and also reflect on what they have already done, as they may have forgotten. We ask families to write on calendars when they are likely to visit. This is great for residents to see and look forward to. Of course, activities may include sports clubs, luncheon clubs, etc. It is important that the interests and hobbies of the individual are considered, as well as their capabilities. For example, we have sensory trails in the garden or sensory quizzes if people have hearing loss or poor vision. Activities are also provided in braille or large print and in different languages.

Question:

How does the individual usually spend their day?

Part C
Activities of Daily Living

10.
Mobility

"Put your heart, mind and soul into even the smallest acts. This is the secret of success."

SWAMI SIVANANDA

For many of us, walking is one of those activities we do without thinking, simply by putting one foot in front of the other. But when you are dealing with a person who is ageing or frail there are other factors to consider. Firstly, older people have a gait and posture that is unique to them, which they have developed over time. This alters balance when they walk, and they learn what makes them *feel* safe and not necessarily what *is* the safest way to move or transfer. Illness or disease may also affect their mobility. As we age, our bones become extremely fragile and are therefore susceptible to falling and fractures.

Other factors that can affect mobility and balance include a stroke, anaemia and medication, so it is important to understand an individual's medical history. It may be helpful to make an appointment for them to see their GP to review them. With their consent, the GP can inform you of any diagnoses made. If someone has recurrent falls, there may be a medical reason for it, including a drop in blood pressure, an irregular heartbeat or impaired vision, as well as those previously mentioned. Try encouraging the individual to have regular check-ups with either their GP or practice nurse.

It is important to observe a person's mobility in their own environment and see how they mobilise. Note if they use sticks, a Zimmer frame or they lean on furniture that is carefully placed to assist them when getting around. Another good indicator for balance and strength is to observe how an individual gets up from a chair. If they use both arms on the armrests to lift themselves up, they are considered to have good strength. Alternatively, if they try to stand up without using their arms to hold onto the armrests or table or struggle to coordinate the task, it provides some indication of their frailty score. Keeping active and completing regular exercises encourages better balance, mobility and muscle. There are many videos online to re-educate people how to get up from a chair safely and these are helpful for chair-based exercises.

Assessing someone's mobility is not as easy as it seems. I cared for a lady in her nineties who refused to walk, although she was capable of doing so. One day I informed her that I needed to complete a risk assessment and review her mobility. She duly obliged after lots of persuasion, walking very confidently but slowly with a Zimmer frame. When I asked her why she declined to walk for the care staff, she smiled at me and replied, "Why walk when you can be wheeled?" Of course, this is an isolated case, but it is important to acknowledge that some people rely on others too much.

Mental agility also influences the physical abilities of a person as they age. We had a gentleman in the care home who could not walk during the day without the assistance of two staff either side of him and a Zimmer frame in front to lean on. He had Parkinson's Disease and early-stage dementia and would shake and be unsteady, but he wanted his independence so did not want to use a wheelchair. He was unstable at times and easily distracted and so did not always focus on where he was going. However, at night between 3 am and 5 am he could often be found dressed, out in the lounge without his frame and unaccompanied. When staff tried to encourage him to walk back to his room, he would start shaking and stumbling again, as though he had forgotten how to walk. It was unbelievable how subconsciously he walked unaided, when he didn't have distractions, yet when people informed him of where he was and brought him back to the moment, he almost did not believe them and would lose his confidence. The agitation caused him to stiffen up his body and lose the ability to mobilise without assistance and guidance. This could possibly be attributed to the stillness of the night, enabling him to concentrate, without any distractions caused by noise or visual disturbances. While it was challenging for the night staff several times a week, it was also a unique opportunity to witness someone regress back to a time when they were more independent, and it gave him a significant sense of well-being.

Although it was the middle of the night, it was important that staff did not disturb him. At this time, he was a proud man getting ready for his day independently. It was a shame that later in the day he had no recollection of it.

It is important to assess if an individual requires aids within the home environment to maintain their independence. There are an increasing number of mobility shops around, and social services will also have information of where to source mobility aids. These may be simple but effective, including a rail in the bathroom or by the bedside, a commode or raised toilet seat. An occupational therapist (OT) can also offer an assessment and guidance on all aids or adaptations required for an older frail person and they can be contacted via the individual's GP.

Question:

How well does the individual mobilise?

11.
Falls

"Do not judge me by my successes, judge me by how many times I fell down and got back up again."

NELSON MANDELA

Falls are one of the most common problems older people encounter, and recurrent falls can indicate that someone's health is deteriorating, hence a chapter dedicated entirely to falling and the risks of falls. However, as people age they actually accept it as a consequence of getting older.

Research shows that common factors that increase the risk of falling include being female, over the age of 80, on more than five medications and a lack of exercise.

The outcome of a fall can range from a minor cut or bruising to a loss of confidence, a severe fracture and a subsequent hospital admission for an operation. Therefore, health-care professionals and carers should be proactive in trying to reduce the likelihood of a fall. The risk can never be completely eliminated, but there are interventions that can assist the independence of someone who is ageing and reduce the incidences of falls or the serious impact of a fall.

It is also important to discover why an individual is falling. It could be due to a number of reasons, such as low blood pressure, a blood deficiency or an underlying illness or disease. It is advisable for people to have regular check-ups with their GP or practice nurse to rule some of these out.

Observe the individual's mobility in their own environment and note if they use furniture to mobilise. If they use a stick or frame/walker, do they use it appropriately. Some people who have a Zimmer frame lift the wheels off the ground instead of pushing it along (or they often forget to use it). Within a home environment there can be potential trip hazards that can cause a fall, including rugs, uneven steps (indoors or outdoors) and clutter. There are simple steps to address these, which will make it safer for the individual to live and will put them at less risk of a fall or fracture; for example, handrails at appropriate places in the home to support mobility, a riser/recliner chair and secure footwear.

There are, however, some individuals who will remain fiercely independent and will decline any advice or support, wishing to do their own thing. We admitted a lady who'd had over 15 falls in the year prior to her admission and made no issue of her falls. When asked what had happened at home and how she'd managed to get up, she replied, "I just pressed my alarm and the ambulance crew would get me up."

It became routine for her, as she knew help would always come. What she never considered was the cost of the ambulance and the crew each time and the impact on other emergencies that required their urgent assistance. The number of falls prompted her family to review her care needs and she was admitted to our care home.

However, there could have been a review by the falls team in the community, an occupational therapist assessment of the home environment and a medication review prior to the decision to send her to a care home. I also believe loneliness was an influencing factor. This lady lived alone and had become more isolated as she became frailer. She was severely obese and her mobility was restricted, but she knew people would come when she used the alarm bell and transfer her to hospital to check she had not severely injured herself. She would remain an in-patient for 24–48 hours. Each time she would have blood tests and usually an X-ray to check for underlying causes for the fall or serious injury.

Through no fault of the emergency services, their prompt response created the expectation this lady had that "someone will get me up each time I fall", and the lady failed to take any responsibility for this. Her doctor or community nurses should have involved her and discussed with her and her family the number of falls, why she fell and asked her if she wanted support. Since her admission, the care home has adapted her bedroom for her needs and she has been reviewed by her GP and the Falls Prevention Team, who provided her with exercises and a new frame to mobilise. She has fallen since admission, but it has reduced to between two and four times annually. She had a stroke and a weak knee and this does impact on her mobility.

We admitted another lady, over 90 years old, who had osteoporosis and a history of previous fractures. Our assessments proved she was deemed at high risk of falling and at high risk of sustaining a fracture if she fell. The home, along with her family, tried everything to reduce the risk of her falling and injuring herself. She used a Zimmer frame to mobilise and had bars placed next to her bed, by her toilet and beside her chair, but she rarely used them because she did not want to. She wanted to carry on the same way she had done for years. Even when it was explained to her that she was at high risk of falling and breaking her hip, she would reply, "I don't care."

For a further two years she remained independent in our care home and she was right: she did not fall. However, staff could see she was becoming frailer and stumbling when she mobilised, yet she still declined any support. Sadly, despite her family and staff members' efforts, she did sustain a fall and it was heartbreaking to see her lying on the floor in pain. Eventually, she accepted the use of a stick to mobilise. She was advised to use a Zimmer frame but she declined, stating it was only for old, sick people (she was 94!). This lady was fiercely independent and had the mental capacity to make her own decisions. Her family would become exasperated with her, as she would decline any offers of advice they provided. From her point of view, she wasn't worried about risks. She was more concerned with remaining independent and doing her own thing in her own way After all, she had been doing it for over 90 years.

One question I always ask when assessing someone for admission is how many falls they have had in the last six months in comparison to the six months previous to that. It provides some insight into the frailty of the individual. It is also worth noting whether the individual still takes part in any exercise during the week, as exercise helps keep older people agile, and even those who cannot mobilise can benefit from simple chair-based exercises

– which some leisure centres or community halls offer – to stretch their muscles and maintain balance.

There is always an element of risk when looking after someone who is older. The best one can do is seek the right support and advice from a professional.

Again, the prevalence of technology has enabled the independence of people, particularly in their own homes: sensor mats in beds or on the floor beside the bed (they alarm when someone has moved), or connected devices such as Amazon Echo, which understands verbal commands to turn lights on/off. There are other simple measures that can be taken to prevent someone over stretching, such as using a commode in the bedroom instead of walking along a corridor or reviewing the layout of a room. A good bedside lamp and sensory lights are also very beneficial.

Question:

How many times has the person fallen in the last year?

12.
Nutrition and Hydration

*"When I was young, I admired clever people.
Now I am old, I admire kind people."*

ABRAHAM J. HESCHEL

Good nutrition is essential for everyone, but as we age, activity levels decline and metabolism slows. It has a huge impact on a person's well-being. Eating and drinking is a part of everyday life, so as adults we do not tend to think about the process of eating and drinking. We usually eat when we are hungry and drink when we are thirsty. Of course, there is a routine to it: we have breakfast soon after waking up, lunch halfway through the day and dinner in the evening. People don't often view eating and drinking as a separate activity; it just naturally becomes part of their daily lives. Even as adults our well-being can affect our eating habits. When feeling low or at times of stress, people feel they want to consume everything or just do not feel like eating.

For many older people (and I mean those generally over the age of 80), eating becomes an important part of the day. I have found it is either something they really look forward to and enjoy or is a time of struggle or angst that has to be encountered every day. It has been more noticeable over the past ten years that more older people are being admitted to our care home either underweight or malnourished. After all, it is well documented that malnutrition affects a significant proportion of the older population living alone in the UK. The cause of this can include memory loss, dysphagia (difficulty swallowing), underlying disease or poor oral health. They may also become deficient in nutrients and minerals or a combination of these factors.

It is important to note if you think the person you care for has lost weight, as many cannot always recognise it themselves. Look for signs of weight loss, such as loose-fitting clothes, poorly fitting dentures, lethargy, gaunt appearance or weak, broken nails. Often weight loss occurs over time and is unintentional. It is important that the individual is reviewed by their GP, as there could also be a medical reason why this is occurring. How you approach this is important, as the individual may not recognise they have a problem. It is better to advise them to have a routine check-up with their GP, who should check their body mass index (BMI) and possibly arrange routine bloods to be taken.

Many people who live alone enjoy cooking for themselves, but equally there are many who find it a chore. Add frailty and difficulty standing, poor dexterity or lethargy, and you can see why some older people prefer convenience foods. These are often quicker and easier to make. Shopping and cooking can be difficult for someone who has a physical disability. It is also easier and cheaper to buy tinned foods, which will have a longer shelf life, so check fridges and kitchen cupboards for supplies and sell-by dates.

The ability to consume three nutritious meals daily creates many challenges as people become older adults. After all, as we get older our bodies change, and what our body wants and likes also changes.

We had one lady who routinely woke early for a cup of tea at 5 am. She then went back to bed and woke for another cup at 6 am, followed by her cereal, then toast with another cup of tea. Any unexpected change in this routine would cause her to be agitated throughout the day and she would sometimes not eat any lunch due to this. Another lady would eat breakfast and then pick at her lunch and supper, so at night we had to leave her a wrapped sandwich for when she became hungry. We tried to alter this and encourage her to nibble during the day, but she had created this routine for herself at home over five years prior to coming into the care home.

We all develop a relationship with food, sometimes healthy and sometimes unhealthy. Therefore, it is important to establish an individual's habits in relation to food preferences and allergies, how often they eat and where they prefer to eat.

As part of our admission process, residents are weighed and asked what weight they think they are and whether they enjoy food/meals. Remarkably, some do not notice they have lost weight, even when it is five to ten per cent of their body weight.

Helpful Tips for Nutrition:

- Encourage a variety of foods.
- Try and eat with them; it can be lonely eating on your own.
- Play the radio or music in the background.
- Give people time to eat; they should not be rushed.
- Suggest an oral health check.
- Give small amounts that are easy to pick up (fork or finger foods).
- Have a supply of snacks/nibbles between meals.
- Have a drink available as this softens food to aid swallowing

Malnutrition

Malnutrition can occur very quickly in people as they age, yet it can remain undetected. People often imagine someone malnourished as extremely thin or emaciated and living in a third world country, yet there are thousands of people living in the UK who are under-nourished. Fortunately, it can be reversed and can also be prevented. The consequences of malnourishment for many is that it can also lead to infections and delay in recovery from illness, as well as increased hospital admission and length of stay.

Recently, I visited a blind resident who had been admitted to hospital with severe low blood pressure and kidney failure. At that time she had been in hospital for nearly six weeks and I reviewed her documentation as she was deemed fit for discharge. I noted she had lost almost 20 lbs in weight since admission. I asked the nurse on duty if this was being addressed and was shocked that it had not been noticed. I understand that many people are not weighed in hospital and that the priority was to treat her blood pressure and kidney failure, but this lady was visibly wasting away. She had no energy reserves to support her recovery. In hospital, dehydration can be addressed with intravenous fluids but poor nutrition is not so easy to detect, unless someone is monitoring it.

I have noticed over the years that an older person's nutritional intake has an impact on their well-being, socialisation and energy levels, and often our care staff and relatives of residents notice the positive change in their loved one once they have been in the home a few weeks and are eating regular nutritious meals. In the last 25 years, everyone who has been prescribed laxatives in our home has had them discontinued due to regular, nutritious food and hydration. There is no reason why this should not be the case in the community as well.

Hydration

Adequate hydration is also vitally important in a person's overall well-being and health. On average a person should drink eight glasses of fluid daily, but this is challenging for people who are frail and lack an appetite. One major factor to consider is a fear of being incontinent or having to rush to the toilet and not arriving in time. An unfamiliar environment can cause anxiety and cause a person undue stress, as they do not know where the toilets are or are too frightened or ashamed to raise the issue.

If someone is reluctant to drink because they are worried about incontinence, it may be worth visiting a place before to familiarise them with the location of the toilets, parking as near to the entrance as possible and sitting near toilets that are clearly signed.

Fluids are also important to help prevent constipation, which is very common in older people. Medication for constipation should be avoided if possible, as it can often cause wind and gut spasms, which can be painful. There are alternative ways to encourage fluids, such as ice, gravy, ice lollies, soup and fruit. A variety of drinks should also be considered. We often use cartons of fruit juice or smoothies, as people find these a fresh alternative to squash and lemonade, and they are small, handy cartons that can be carried and opened when desired.

Question:

Has the person lost weight in the last year?

13.
Personal Care

"Being vulnerable is the only way to allow your heart to feel true pleasure."

BOB MARLEY

Personal care involves washing, bathing, showering and dressing. It also includes going to the bathroom. It creates a routine to help at the start of the day and also prepares us for a peaceful night. Most have a preference for a bath or shower but there are many who prefer to opt for a daily wash or freshen up and intermittent baths or showers. Washing and dressing can be so tiring as someone becomes frail, so a quick freshen up may be preferable.

Bathrooms are considered high-risk areas for people who are frail, as the floor can become slippery and stepping into a shower or bath requires good balance and dexterity. It is important to assess the risk of falling in the bathroom and seek help for aids, such as a non-slip mat, bars to hold on to and a shower seat.

Buttons and zips also start to become an issue, and, therefore, loose clothing becomes ideal. Plain tops can be rejuvenated with a scarf or brooch. People prefer to wear familiar clothing rather than new clothing. One lady preferred to wear the same undergarments, which were threadbare, but she remembered buying them and she said she always felt comfortable in them. Had we not discussed it with her, they would definitely have been thrown out as her family bought new ones. They were important to her, so staff looked after them as if they were new. It is important to recognise that older people feel safe with familiar clothing, as they are filled with memories and familiarity, just like photographs.

People should be encouraged to wear make-up, brush their own hair and wear jewellery if it makes them feel good. Usually, you can notice a slight decline in someone when they lose interest in washing or their appearance, so it is worth looking out for this. We had one lovely lady in our care home who deteriorated with a suspected chest infection and the ambulance was called. Despite being breathless and very unwell, she insisted on applying her bright-red lipstick before the ambulance crew arrived. It was so important to her that she always looked her best regardless of the situation.

Going to the Toilet

Sometimes even the simplest of tasks can be difficult and one such endeavour is going to the bathroom. It is a difficult subject to discuss, as it is not something people wish to consider and is so personal and intimate, but it is important to recognise the impact ageing has on all aspects of the body. There is also support to help assess the layout of the home and bathrooms by an occupational therapist, and via the GP and a continence specialist to offer advice and solutions to any continence issues.

As our bodies get older our muscles naturally become weaker and many often find they lose the ability to retain urine and need to go to the bathroom more frequently. Certain conditions can also have an impact on an older person's behaviour and attitude to going to the toilet, particularly if they have a condition that affects their bowel or bladder, such as irritable bowel syndrome, diverticulitis or a prolapsed uterus. It is important that care providers, family and friends acknowledge any condition or illness that may influence an older person's toilet habits and assist them in planning their care needs sensitively to avoid any embarrassment or distress. This can be particularly evident when going on a car journey. It is wise to plan regular toilet breaks so the individual has the opportunity to go to the bathroom without having to be asked.

Even though someone may be perfectly capable of going to the bathroom independently during the day, it can be very different at night. Some individuals may prefer a commode or urinal by their bed, so they do not have to walk to the bathroom, as there is an increased risk of falls and incontinence. Some may take medication for high blood pressure and this could affect their balance at night.

Leaving a night light (or touch-sensitive light) in the room or hallway is beneficial.

Access to a bathroom is a huge concern for older people, particularly within a social situation, including location and the availability of aids to assist them once they are in the bathroom, such as a raised toilet seat or handles for support. Many people refrain from visiting a bathroom when they are out socially for fear of not reaching it in time or of causing a fuss and upsetting the person they are spending time with. It is important that the companion looks out for any signs of agitation but also encourages the individual to attend the bathroom prior to a car journey. Washing hands can be difficult when using a Zimmer frame or walker, so toiletries, including wet wipes, could be useful.

As mentioned in the previous chapter, people reduce their fluid intake for fear of being incontinent and any subsequent dehydration may lead to other problems, including urinary tract infections. In care establishments there is always a constant battle, as it is difficult to persuade older people to stay hydrated and drink more because they have a genuine fear of being incontinent and of waking up several times during the night. They would prefer to risk developing a urine infection but have a better night's sleep and remain continent. This is less embarrassing or demeaning for them.

Incontinence pads should be considered if someone finds it difficult to reach the bathroom in time. It is referred to as stress incontinence. Assessment by a trained practitioner can advise on equipment and pads and they can also be available free on the National Health Service (NHS), so it is worth asking the GP for a referral to the continence nurse. They can also advise on eating and drinking habits and exercises to strengthen the pelvic floor muscles.

Bowels

As people age, they develop a habit or routine regarding their bowel movements. It is important to try to maintain their usual routine, as this will cause them less stress. But there are other factors that influence bowel habits; illness, stress, dehydration, hot weather and medication can all influence bowel habits.

Unfortunately, some older people become so fixated on opening their bowels daily that if they fail to do this, they will try to self-evacuate, and it is important to recognise that class and wealth have no influence in this well-known habit of older people. It is difficult to approach, as the individual can become embarrassed and refute any accusation that they have self-evacuated. Therefore, it must be approached with sensitivity and compassion. Eating a nutritious balanced meal with fruit and fibre and maintaining hydration is important and impacts on toileting practices.

Question:

Does the person manage any personal care themselves?

14.
Sexuality

"Love and compassion are necessities, not luxuries. Without them humanity cannot survive."

DALAI LAMA

Traditionally, sexuality has been an area that most health-care professionals find difficult to approach. It can feel uncomfortable asking an older person about their sexuality or sexual preferences, but it can be approached in a sensitive manner. It may be more comfortable finding out about personal space, comfort and relationships: who is important in the person's life? If care is being arranged at home, it is important to understand the person's attitude to carers of the opposite sex and to discuss this with the care provider. Encourage the person to ask questions and explore their feelings about it.

The word 'sexuality' covers a myriad of thoughts, feelings and ideas and can mean something different to everyone. When supporting an individual with their care needs, it is important that personal care and sexuality is discussed in context and that a broader view is taken, as it involves different aspects of need, physical comfort, love and support. Sexuality can be influenced by life experiences, gender, personality and attitude. A discussion about sexuality (or needs) should be approached with sensitivity and in confidence at an appropriate time.

However, it can be a difficult subject to approach with older people. In care homes staff try to determine a person's attitude towards carers of the opposite sex or other residents within the communal areas. For example, an individual may have a stoma requiring assistance. Some do not wish care staff of the opposite sex to care for their personal needs. Everyone has a right to be treated with dignity and to be supported how they wish, with any care needs they have, and this includes sexuality.

Within care provision it is important that people in care are supported to express who is important in their lives and any personal needs they may have. They will be informed about any communal areas, particularly bathrooms, and if they have a male or female carer to support them in their care needs. Fortunately, attitudes are changing and there is now a recognition of sexual orientation and people are encouraged to express themselves how they wish. We had a lady in her nineties who never married and informed us she had never had a boyfriend. She was shocked at the idea of a man helping her wash and seeing her undressed. At first only female staff tended to her needs, but as she became more familiar with male staff and interacted with them during activities and at lunch she changed her opinion. She got to know them and built a professional relationship built on trust. Often older people feel more relaxed when they know someone is available, ready to help them regardless of their gender.

Many care providers promote diversity and equality, believing that each individual is unique and should be treated with respect. This includes sexual orientation or preferences, and therefore it should be discussed.

The Power of Touch

I have observed that even the most strong-willed individuals can be sentimental, often at times of distress or frailty. In our care home, residents can become emotional and often reach out to touch their carer's hand or lean their head on their carer's shoulder. It can be quite a tender response when someone is reminiscing about their life or loved ones. While it is not openly encouraged, touching someone's hand or giving them a hug can be a natural response to demonstrate thoughtfulness and shows the individual that you care and understand how they are feeling. It is an important time to be dignified and sensitive to an individual's emotions and overall well-being.

Relationships and sexuality in social care

The regulatory body for health and social care providers, the Care Quality Commission (CQC), published guidance on relationships and sexuality in social care. It highlighted that people may feel judged by those providing their care. It is important to facilitate a holistic approach to care, so everyone understands the importance of maintaining relationships and expressing sexuality. This includes all sexuality, particularly anyone who may have experienced discrimination or prejudice in their lives. There should be no discrimination against love, regardless of who is involved.

Question:

Does the person have a relationship/companion or sexual needs?

15.
Sleeping

"Try to be a rainbow in someone's cloud."

MAYA ANGELOU

Everyone needs a good night's sleep regardless of their age. Our bodies need plenty of sleep in order to function efficiently. Many cite seven to nine hours a night but it is more important for everyone to listen to their own body clock and establish what is right for them. As we get older and experience changes in our body and mind, many suffer from insomnia caused by medical conditions, medication (particularly polypharmacy), dementia, depression and loneliness. It can also present itself as waking frequently during the night, waking up very early in the morning or feeling exhausted during the day. A good night's sleep is essential to enable older people to function well and remain in good health.

Medication can also cause drowsiness, so it is worth asking the GP to review not only the medication but the time of day it is taken. For example, it is feasible to take certain blood pressure tablets and sedation medication before bedtime and diuretics in the daytime, preferably in the morning, as these are stimulants.

Stress can also cause insomnia and this can be triggered by a traumatic event, such as the death of a spouse. We once cared for a lady who had been burgled at night when she lived at home. She lay in bed pretending to be asleep and the burglar took her jewellery and, fortunately, ran out of the house and she was unharmed. However, this prompted her admission to the care home and she would often wake up several times a night, as she was haunted by the figure. Leaving a light on and her door ajar acted as a reminder that staff were around during the night and she had a call bell if she felt frightened and needed support.

Night-time can be the most difficult part of the day and so people may have the television or radio playing until their bodies force them to go to sleep. One lady who lived on her own found it the loneliest time and would have the television on just to hear noise. She was frightened of living alone ever since her husband passed away.

Routine

Another lady wakes several times during the night to go to the bathroom, starts her daily routine at 4.30 am, washing and dressing. She has a cup of tea at 5 am and waits until 7 am to have her breakfast. Staff have tried to encourage her to have a lie-in until 6 am, but she says she cannot. She used to be a bank clerk and would walk to the bank and this habit has remained into her late nineties.

Boredom itself can cause people to sleep more. If someone has no stimulation or regular pattern to their day, they can become bored and get into the habit of napping during the day. After retirement, and with the onset of physical ailments, older people can find it more difficult to engage in activities that they used to find enjoyable.

Of course, any break in sleep pattern during the night can cause an individual to sleep for short periods during the day to catch up on hours lost, and this is good for cognitive function, social interaction and memory. This does not necessarily mean returning to the bedroom for a lie down, as many prefer to remain in the comfort of their armchair for a nap. It is important, therefore, to review the type of chair the person is using and an investment in a recliner chair may be a wise choice.

Helpful Tips for Quality Sleep

Age UK have published a document entitled 'Healthy Living: Maintaining a Healthy Mind and Body', which suggests useful considerations to help an individual get enough good-quality sleep. These included:

- cutting down on daytime naps
- going to bed at the same time each night

- not eating or drinking alcohol too close to bedtime
- reducing the amount of caffeine during the day and trying decaf tea or coffee
- getting up and doing something for half an hour if the person can't get to sleep before going back to bed.

Question:

How much sleep does the person get each day?

16.
Dying

"Our most cruel failure in how we treat the sick and the aged is the failure to recognise that they have priorities beyond merely being safe and living longer."

ATUL GAWANDE

Life and death are a part of living, but as a lady once asked me, "At what point does a person stop living and start dying?" I felt this lady had posed a very interesting question and one which I had not considered before. However, after the recent death of my own mum, I recognise the huge impact that losing a loved one has on an individual. Now imagine reaching 90 years of age, having lost both parents, your spouse and one or two siblings. There are less family and friends to socialise or interact with and you are dealing with frailty and possible illness. This is the reality of many people who enter care homes. Many do not want to go into a care home, as it is perceived as the waiting room for the inevitable, final destination. It is understandable for people to view each day as tiresome and not meaningful. The world they are currently living in appears more alien to the one they grew up in. However, the reality of modern care homes is that often with the right social stimulation, company of others and good care, people experience a better and more meaningful quality of life in their later years. It is fair to say that many people fear death and often avoid talking about it, but it is an inevitable part of life. Even within a caring profession I understand why people avoid talking about illness, ageing and death.

By understanding this dilemma, care staff approach an admission to a care home with sensitivity and an awareness of what the individual is going through emotionally and physically.

When looking after someone who is vulnerable, delicate questions need to be asked and wishes discussed, at the right time. People can deteriorate quickly but by having their wishes documented, family and health-care professionals can deliver dignified care in the right environment, as chosen by the individual.

Advanced care plans (ACPs) and living wills can determine an individual's preferences for the care they wish and do not wish to receive at particular times. This includes refusing treatment, even if it leads to the individual's death. It is essential that the person is given time to consider what they want and are not rushed into any hasty decisions.

It may be worth discussing how the person perceives their quality of life, their overall health and what assistance they feel they need. From this discussion one can evaluate the individual's understanding of the impact of their age, illness or any frailty they may have. ACP's set out a person's preferences and thoughts about future care if they become ill, require invasive treatment or resuscitation.

It is difficult to talk to someone about death and dying but it is important to ask sensitive questions at the right time and discuss their wishes if they suddenly become unwell.

No one needs to make any immediate decisions, but it does give the person an opportunity to talk about how they feel they are getting on in life and to start thinking about what they would like to happen at a time when they may become incapacitated and unable to make decisions. It is easier to go through it at a time when the individual has capacity and is relatively fit and able to make decisions.

Questions to Consider

If you were to become unwell:

- what do you want/not want to happen to you?
- who would you wish to be involved in any decisions about you?
- would you like to go to hospital or stay at home?
- would you want to receive all treatment and care (including invasive procedures)?

- would you want to receive non-invasive treatment and care?
- would you want to be resuscitated if your heart was to stop?

Of course, as people age they become more aware of their own mortality and think about death and dying in private. There is usually a particular time for each individual when they no longer relate to the length of time they have left but rather the quality of the time they have left. This became more evident to me while caring for a particular lady (mentioned earlier) who when staff would say "See you in the morning" would reply, "I hope not dear; I just want to close my eyes and not open them again." Staff found this peculiar and felt uncomfortable when she said it. After all, she was in good health, was well cared for and had a loving family.

Intrigued, I asked her why she repeated these words each night to the care staff. She was very clear and astute when she explained to me that her poor daughter would visit her nearly every day and had recently become a grandmother herself but she felt she tied her daughter down. "She should live her own life and not worry about me." She continued to explain that she had led a happy life but she felt that at 98, with limited mobility and agility, life wasn't enjoyable and she just felt she *existed*. I tried to convince her that she was still an active lady who participated in events within the home, to which she replied that she did it and enjoyed those times, but inside it wasn't enough. I remember this being a light-bulb moment for me as a care manager because it forced me to view life from her perspective. When I evaluated the quality of her life and looked at how active she had been up until her eighties – she played tennis, was driving and attended social clubs, but then illness interfered with her daily life – I could understand why she felt the way she did. I could see that she participated and enjoyed the activities but this enjoyment was limited to brief moments. In other words, she was experiencing more time unengaged in solitude than engaged with others.

I listened to a debate on the radio about whether the family of a dying person should allow a distant relative or friend to visit them, particularly if they had not seen the dying person for a few years. One listener explained that he did not want his cousin to visit his dad because he had never visited him when he was well, so why should he bother now just because he was dying? Another listener explained that he did not want relatives "coming out of the woodwork" to visit a dying family member, as it seemed inappropriate because they had not seen them for over a decade.

Although I appreciate their points of view, the situation should not be about what they think, but more appropriately, what would the dying person want to happen. This became evident to me while caring for a lady who was dying. She had not seen her brother in over 40 years. In fact, no one knew she even had a brother until we received a phone call from him out of the blue. He had heard through extended family members that she was dying and he wanted to come and see her. Of course, we explained we would need to ask the lady and her family. The family were adamant he should not be allowed to visit, as they had not spoken since they had fallen out many years ago. I asked the lady herself if she would like her brother to visit and she replied that she *did* want to see him.

At first they were polite to each other, catching up with small talk about their families, and then she asked me if I could go and get some tea for them both, which I did. Upon my return they were quietly talking and listening to each other and the atmosphere was very calm. After two hours he left and I returned to the room and the lady appeared content and serene, as though a huge weight had been lifted from her shoulders. I never asked what they had talked about but I could see she genuinely appeared content. It transpired that they had reconciled their differences that had kept them apart for so many years. It created closure for them both.

At first her family were very disapproving of her brother appearing out of the blue, but I was able to reassure them that on reflection it was comforting for her and she had benefited from the visit. It was a beautiful experience to have witnessed.

When people become aware that they are reaching a time when they may not live for very long, their attitudes and perspectives can alter. More recently, people are creating bucket lists to complete before they die or are recording videos/blogs of their thoughts and feelings, mapping how they are coping living with an illness. Many appear to accept the inevitable, relax and enjoy the simplicity of life. Their senses become heightened: smell, sound, touch. They often reflect on how grateful they are for the care and attention provided by everyone.

Dignity in care is extremely important, particularly during end-of-life care. One exercise we performed in our care home was to create a dignity tree, where each resident, their relatives, members of staff and visitors to the home wrote down on a paper leaf what dignity meant to them. Most wrote "Treat me like an individual", "Respect my privacy" or "Ask me what I want". One lady wrote "Look after me when I am dead". I was so shocked by this, as all the other comments reflected on the present time. I asked her privately what she had meant by her words and she explained that she felt that no one would attend her funeral, as she had no family or friends, and she had one wish, which was that her dog, who had passed away several years before, would be buried with her. (He had been cremated and his ashes were in a sealed wooden box in her wardrobe).

About 18 months later, this lady died due to ill health and her words never left me. I, along with another member of staff, attended her burial. One of us read a passage from the Bible and the other read a poem that the resident had written during a poetry activity session a few years earlier. We ensured that her beloved dog was buried with her. I feel extremely proud that we carried out her wishes and gave her a dignified burial.

Noting religious or personal beliefs ensures that any religious representatives may attend when the person requests. Even those with no known religion may wish to receive a blessing when they are extremely unwell. This can be an emotional time, so it should be respected.

End of Life

At this time, advanced care plans are followed and the wishes of the person respected. People are given the opportunity to reflect on memories and times that were important to them. Some choose to have particular music or noises played in their rooms, fresh flowers, favourite perfume, particular blanket or dressing gown draped over their bed, dimmed lights or a picture of loved ones within easy view. It is an extremely personal and bespoke time for everyone involved.

End of life in the community has been transformed, with GP practices, district nurses and palliative care professionals supporting those who choose to remain at home during the end of their lives. There are various organisations and charities who also provide support and advice for both the individual and their family.

Question:

Do you know what the person wants if they become unwell?

17.
Dementia and Memory Loss

"They may forget what you said but they will not forget how you made them feel."

HEATHER LOUISE

Dementia is a very debilitating disease but understanding what it is and how it affects the person can ensure that the individual maintains a life full of enrichment and receives the right care support. Memory loss is the most common sign of dementia: forgetting names and events or repeating the same fact several times. This is commonly known about dementia but it can also cause a change in behaviour, cognitive function and reasoning. The impact can affect all aspects of daily life for those living with it.

When someone becomes aware that they cannot remember simple names or where they left their keys, wallet, etc., they can become embarrassed and socially introverted, as they do not want others to notice. Living with dementia is very challenging both for the individual and their family or friends. It is important that if the individual you are caring for develops signs or symptoms of dementia or memory loss, you should seek help for them straight away. The GP can refer them to a memory clinic.

Memory loss affects people differently and can present in a variety of ways. Some merely forget they have explained something and repeat it but others can become suspicious, accusing others of moving their personal belongings or of theft, when in fact they have moved items and money themselves. I have cared for people who were convinced people had stolen their property, when in fact, staff have found money or jewellery in pillowcases, drawers, tissue boxes and within the pages of books.

People with dementia often prefer routine, as they feel safer and more comfortable, so a plan of how the individual likes to spend their day would be beneficial. Note what makes them happy or what activities they particularly enjoy. Distraction therapy at the right moment may draw attention away from a challenging situation or discussion that is causing the individual distress.

A memory box is a wonderful tool when a person with dementia becomes distressed. It can be personalised to contain items of interest and memory for them, including old photographs, a prayer book, their favourite perfume, a personal tapestry or knitting. One lady possessed her father's whistle, as he was a train conductor, and her box contained an old powder puff she used during wartime. These boxes are great for reminiscence sessions and help people with memory loss focus on objects that they can relate to and talk about, providing comfort and support. Calendars, notepads and post-it notes, as visual stimulants, are also very useful ways of giving people independence.

Music therapy is a fantastic tool to aid someone with dementia, as music affects a different part of the brain, which retains the memory of melodies. Noting any music genres or particular songs that a person enjoys or holds a special memory of can promote their well-being. If I had to choose two songs, they would be Abba's 'Dancing Queen', which reminds me of nights out during my nurse training in London, and 'When a Child is Born', sung by Charlie Pride. When I was five years of age, I went into hospital to have my tonsils removed, and this was the song my mum dedicated to me on the hospital radio. Every time I hear them played, they not only remind me of those times but they make me emotionally regress and experience those times again.

When people think of dementia, they often think about the mental ability of an individual. However, often with an impairment of the brain there is also a change in the physical ability of an individual, such as their peripheral vision or balance. Changes can become impaired over time, so observe for minor changes.

I cared for one lady who had a diagnosis of dementia and retained a good memory but could not negotiate the act of sitting in a chair. She would often sit on the arm of the chair or almost on the lap of the person in the adjacent chair. She would walk to the chair using her Zimmer frame, but once she got there she could not remember how to sit down. Our activity coordinator spent many hours with her relearning how to get up and sit down from a chair safely.

We also cared for a lady who would often eat a huge two-course dinner and within 20 minutes of finishing would tell visitors that she had not eaten all day and was being starved. We would give her the meal and then leave a note beside her stating which meal it was: for example, "This is your lunch of chicken casserole, mashed potatoes, carrots and green beans." The pattern of placing the card next to her offered her reassurance.

The Alzheimer's Society has provided helpful factsheets for individuals and family members about living with dementia. Some helpful hints in caring for an individual with memory loss include:

- asking yourself whether it really matters if the person remembers a recent conversation or event – forcing the matter can make things worse
- setting up a regular routine – this can make it easier for the person to remember what is going to happen during the day
- encouraging them to use a diary or journal to record things that have happened – pictures and words are useful tools, as they can be used to remind the person what they have done and as a conversation starter
- including cues and prompts, and trying to give context, instead of asking vague questions: for example, "It must be a while since breakfast. Are you hungry?" rather than "Have you had breakfast?"
- considering using reminders such as sticky notes or a wall calendar for one-off tasks, and more permanent reminders for tasks the person does more often, such as keeping a note by the door to remember keys and wallet
- focusing on one thing at a time – giving the person too much information may be overwhelming
- keeping information simple and repeating it often (if necessary)
- reducing distractions, such as background noise
- keeping questions simple and specific: for example, "Do you want tea or coffee?" rather than "What would you like to drink?" – by narrowing down their options, you can help the person make a choice

Communication

When communicating with someone who has dementia, it is important to speak clearly and calmly. Non-verbal communication is also key: respecting personal space, smiling, eye contact and touch. If someone appears confused, do not try to correct them, as this can be more distressing for them. If they become agitated, do not try to pre-empt their answer and answer for them; although performed with good intentions, it does not help the person who is confused. Remain calm and smile for reassurance. Short sentences and closed questions are also helpful, and use visual cues where possible.

If a person is able to make decisions, it is important that they are supported to do so. Capacity can fluctuate, so advice and guidance on the Mental Capacity Act (2005) should be sought to ensure the rights of individuals to allow a balance between risks and the individual's safety. Do not assume someone does not have capacity, even if they have a diagnosis or impairment of the brain, as capacity must always be assumed in the first instance.

Assisted Technology

Over the last decade technology has expanded and has been available to help individuals keep safe and remain independent. It can be used for memory loss, communication difficulties or dementia.

There are many helpful devices around, including:

- pendant alarms – to call for assistance when unwell or after sustaining a fall
- sensor mats – that sense movement and can inform carers when someone with dementia is moving around
- motion sensors – that identify movement and can verbalise a pre-recorded message (such as reminding someone to lock the front door)
- calendar clocks – that help people keep track of the day and date and identify whether it is day or night
- trackers – to use when something is lost

- medication prompts – where times are pre-set and will alarm when someone is due for their medication
- adapted telephones – where instead of remembering numbers, a photo of the family member or friend can be pushed to obtain an instant line to them

The local council should have an assisted-living centre or occupational therapist who can provide advice and information on what is available.

Question:

Does the person have a good memory?

Part D
Support

18.
Funding

"Nowadays people know the price of everything and the value of nothing."

OSCAR WILDE

At some point almost every older person will be dependent on support from another person, whether a neighbour, relative or carer. Researching financial support for social care can be quite complex. The first contact should be the person's GP, to identify any existing illnesses and to discuss care needs. Then contact the local authority's adult social care department for advice and guidance.

It can be very daunting when initially faced with care fees. Many worry about how they will pay for care fees, what happens to their assets and what happens when the money becomes deficient. Paying for care does not only cause stress and strain on the older person but also on those tasked with arranging the care provision. It is essential that people seek financial advice on what care support is needed, where to source the care and the costs involved.

While making plans for the future, I would encourage all adults to write a will. If no will has been written, certain laws and rules dictate how a person's money should be allocated. A will enables the individual to decide what happens to their possessions, property and finances after their death. Later in life, some appoint a power of attorney or joint attorneys, through the Court of Protection. They are identified legally to act on the older person's behalf if they do not have the capacity to act for themselves (Mental Capacity Act 2005). One type of power of attorney relates to financial and property affairs and the other to health and personal welfare. Either family members or a friend may be nominated by the individual to act on their behalf at a time when they may no longer have the capacity to make decisions about their finances or their health. The power of attorney will liaise with health-care professionals to make decisions in the individual's best interest. Too often people sort out their finances but fail to appoint an individual to oversee and help decide their welfare, and this can cause confusion and arguments between family and health-care professionals later on. It is worth ensuring both are considered at the same time.

Financial support is available irrespective of whether individuals choose to stay in their own home. Care costs will vary and will depend on the needs of the individual, their choice of care package and the price of who is providing the care. There are many options that should be considered based on the individual's needs. If they prefer to remain at home for as long as possible, the home could be adapted with suitable furniture such as a raised bed, a commode, handlebars or a stairlift, etc. There have been huge advancements in technology that enable older people to remain in their own homes independently.

Some people choose a stepping-stone approach to care provision, where the home is adapted or a move to sheltered accommodation is made. This is usually beneficial for a few years, but as their needs increase, a higher level of intervention and support is required. Usually, a move to a residential care home or nursing home follows. There is no right pathway to this, as it really is dependent on what the individual needs and, most importantly, wants. They must decide what they would prefer and where is safest for them.

Social services can advise on adaptations to a property and will have a list of approved contractors. They can provide a care assessment to work out what care service an individual may need and make a recommendation. Everyone is entitled to a care assessment. A financial assessment is also worthwhile, to work out entitlement to any financial support. The threshold slightly changes annually but is in the region of £23,000 to £25,000 (2020). With assets over this amount, a person is less likely to qualify for funding support.

However, they may still be entitled to benefits. If an individual has a disability or care needs, they may be entitled to benefits to help meet the cost of care, including Attendance Allowance, Carer's

Allowance and Personal Independence Payment (PIP). Residents of England, Scotland and Wales who have difficulty with everyday tasks may be entitled to make a claim for PIP. (This has replaced the Disability Living Allowance for 16- to 64-year-olds.) There may also be non-selective grants or allowances to consider, such as the winter fuel allowance and council tax reduction.

I would recommend seeking further advice, as funding can be quite complex. An individual may not need to sell their home if they move into a care home, particularly if they have a spouse or a dependent who will remain in the house once they move. There is an option called a deferred payment scheme; a financial advisor or the local authority would provide further advice and guidance.

If someone has no assets, social services may suggest care input while the individual is still able to live at home. This can be paid either by social services directly or to the individual. Their family or advocate can help design the care that the individual wishes, using domiciliary care or a private care provider.

There are many care providers available and the number continues to increase as demand dictates. However, the quality of care provided does vary. I would advise everyone to review the Care Quality Commission website (www.cqc.org.uk) to review inspections of services. Word of mouth is also a powerful tool, so be open to recommendations and use the information as a guide.

Once a care assessment has been completed, contact various care providers and enquire about costs. This varies dramatically from one provider to another and many incur additional costs that are not always visible. It is worth approaching all care providers with the results of a care assessment and have a list of your requirements. Ensure you receive all details written into a contract of care, detailing what exactly is covered. Check the internet for example lists of questions to ask domiciliary and care home providers, as they can be very useful.

If the individual or family/advocate choose to live in a care home that costs more than the local authority would usually expect to pay, they may be asked to meet the difference in cost. This is known as a top-up or third-party agreement. If paying for themselves, the individual has a right to choose which home or care facility they move into, but costs vary considerably and depend on the type of care and the location.

Insurance

A care fee plan is a financial policy offered by some insurers that ensures fees can be paid, regardless of how long the care is required for, in exchange for an upfront lump-sum investment. This could be a preferred option for some. There are care organisations that can advise specifically on funding for later life and will provide an online assessment. In some incidences the NHS may also provide financial support as NHS Continuing Care. This relates to NHS-funded nursing care and covers long-term complex health needs but requires an in-depth assessment by social services, which can be requested.

Question:

Do you need to enquire about funding support?

19.
Conclusion

"Old age has its pleasures, which, though different, are not less than the pleasures of youth."

W. SOMERSET MAUGHAM

Caring for someone else and ensuring they receive the best care and support available is a rewarding experience. Dealing with organisations who provide care support and advice can be challenging, so it may be advisable to share your thoughts and plans with someone else, either a health-care professional or a friend.

The process can be overwhelming at times, but by placing the individual at the heart of all decisions, you will ensure they will receive the right support at the right time. It is inevitable that when dealing with different organisations and someone else's life, there may be mistakes made but this is to be expected. Take your time and make a list of priorities, in the best interests of the individual, acknowledging their preferences and wishes. The outcome is for the individual to feel fulfilled about life and improve their quality of life.

It is also important that you look after yourself as well. When supporting someone else, it is easy to always put them first, but there is a balance between supporting them and looking after your own well-being. At times your feelings will vary. Learn to delegate some tasks, seek advice and guidance and share your experience with others. Carers UK is a wonderful charity that offers support and guidance to people who are caring for others unpaid.

Common Feelings When Caring for Someone:

- Happy
- Lost
- Helpful
- Inexperienced
- Frustrated
- Rejected
- Satisfied

People who reach a certain age are wise, entertaining and have a relaxed attitude about life that we could all benefit from if we spent more time with them and learnt from their experiences of life. Growing old is inevitable, but helping others can have a positive influence on how they experience it.

Older life is also about not taking yourself or life so seriously and not caring about what other people think, so be prepared for honest approaches by the person you care for. It is one advantage of ageing, as experience teaches people what is important and what is not relevant in the complexity of life. People often reflect on their life and reminisce, so embrace the opportunity for the person you care about to impart knowledge and to advise you or your family as the next generation.

Finally, growing old is a state of mind. As you have read this book and I have penned the words, we have both aged a little more. Do you feel any different? I certainly do not. I am still my mother's daughter; I laugh at the silly things in life and I am still passionate about improving the lives and well-being of older people. After all, everyone is unique and important in life, regardless of their age.

Question:

Are you better equipped to support someone who is ageing?

20.
Organisations that Provide Advice and Support

"What is the essence of life? To serve others and to do good."

ARISTOTLE

- Age UK – the national organization for older people (www.ageuk.org.uk)

- Alzheimer's Society – the main charity supporting people and their family with dementia. They offer training for carers and provide ideas for activities for people with dementia (www.alzheimers.org.uk)

- Care Quality Commission – the regulatory body for care providers. They carry out inspections to ensure these services are meeting national standards (www.cqc.org.uk)

- Carer's Trust – the largest charity for carers. It aims to improve services, support and recognition for carers (www.carers.org)

- Carer's UK – provides information about technology and equipment that can support carers in looking after an older person (www.carersuk.org)

- Citizens Advice Bureau – provides free confidential advice to everyone on their rights and responsibilities (www.citizensadvice.org.uk)

- Government website – details on government policy and funding support (www.gov.uk)

- My Home Life led by Age UK in partnership with City University, the Joseph Rowntree Foundation and Dementia UK

Question:

Who do you need to contact for support or advice?

21.
Notes and Questions

*"Do you know what people really want?
Everyone, I mean. Everybody in the world is
thinking: I wish there was just one other person I
could really talk to, who could really understand
me, who'd be kind to me. That's what people
really want, if they're telling the truth."*

DORIS LESSING